# Gluten Free Diet

## HUNDRED GLUTEN

## FREE RECIPES

### BY

### SADIA SANDEELA

# GLUTEN FREE DIET

A gluten-free diet is a diet that is free of all sources of gluten protein. Sources of gluten may include wheat, rye, barley and triticale. This diet is mainly used to treat celiac disease as gluten is being considered to be the source and cause of inflammation in the small intestine. A gluten-free diet has been found to be helpful in the prevention of complications and controlling signs and symptoms associated with this disease.

Majority of all the available wide variety of foods sources do not contain gluten. Therefore diet planning and adaptation need not be difficult to achieve. Basically this diet has been a part of a treatment regimen for celiac disease. Switching to a gluten free diet is not at all that difficult as only few sources of food needed to be avoided in this. Most of the food items are gluten-free naturally and therefore a wide variety of delicious food items are available to be enjoyed in a wide variety of ways.

All natural sources of beans, nuts, seeds, eggs, meat, fish, poultry, dairy, fruits, vegetables and many grains could be enjoyed. Most of the grains and starch groups are naturally free of gluten protein which may include flax, rice, soy, corn, potato, arrowroot, amaranth, buckwheat, millet, quinoa, sorghum, tapioca, teff, etc. Foods that needed to be avoided may include bulgur, farina, durum flour, Graham flour, semolina, spelt, etc. Foods that may contain gluten may include cereals, candies, cakes, pies, breads, beer, croutons, cookies, crackers, French fries, gravies, imitation meat, pastas, salad dressings, soy sauce, sauces, dips, and all processed food products.

Due to gluten intolerance or insensitivity people may choose to go for gluten-free diet. For the general public there is no solid published evidence that supports and suggests that going gluten free is helpful for them. In recent past there has been great interest in gluten-free diet in the general public and consequently the market for gluten-free food products had been expanding progressively. Majority of the people opting for a gluten-free diet had been doing so to find relief from gluten intolerance, sensitivity or allergy.

A word of caution is needed here as unnecessary use of this diet may lead towards food nutrient deficiencies. Wheat flour contains around 12% gluten. Many people consider a gluten-free diet a fad but still there are many who believe that cutting down on many sources of gluten is benefitting them. Gluten-free products have been progressively gaining strength on shelves of super markets and grocery stores. Many people who are not even fully aware of how many benefits this diet has to offer this diet has been part of their dietary trend.

Gluten is a plant protein found mainly in wheat, rye and barley and all food products that contains these food items and helps in maintaining the elasticity of foods during the fermentation phase of food production. It is due to the presence of gluten in bread that we find it chewy. As refined flour is mixed with water it gets more and more elastic during kneading process and this is due to the presence of gluten protein.

Basically a gluten-free diet has a lot to offer if you are suffering from celiac disease, are hypersensitive to gluten or are diagnosed with gluten intolerance. Opting for a gluten free diet may indirectly help you in eliminating many unhealthy food items and food products from your diet that otherwise you are unable to do so e. g. cakes, pastries, cookies, dough nuts and many creamy high in saturated fat and trans-fats food sources of food products. Pure chocolate is gluten free.

But as we are aware that the market for alternatives for gluten-free food products is expanding explosively, this particular protective beneficial element attached with it may get eliminated in due time. If someone is getting benefitted by not eating pastries and cakes today tomorrow they may find gluten-free sources of the same and therefore this beneficial aspect of it will wipe out with time as more gluten-free commercial products starts appearing in the market.

Commercially prepared food products should be avoided in all circumstances because these ontain artificial colors, chemicals and preservatives. Synthetic ingredients have negative effects on overall health and well-being. Consuming a gluten-free diet may help in promoting weight loss if taken in a well-planned and well-balanced manner. For good health benefits, right food items needed to be taken in right proportion.

Keep portion size in mind and be sure to add gluten free starch sources of food items such as sweet potatoes, potatoes, rice, quinoa, corn, etc. Going gluten free may mean saying no to many healthy and nutritious sources of food. Until and unless you are diagnosed with celiac disease or sure of being allergic, sensitive or intolerant to gluten protein you may need not follow this diet as doing so may lead to food nutrient deficiencies.

Gluten rich food sources are also rich sources of many nutrients and cutting down on these foods may mean cutting down on many nutrients. Good dietary planning is needed in order to furnish all the essential nutrients in required quantity on a daily basis to avoid food deficiencies. Meeting the dietary guidelines is a challenge while following this diet.

When you are following a gluten free diet, try to eat home cooked meals instead of eating out. Many gluten free products are available at specialty retailers. Oats can be consumed in moderate amount although these might have been cross contaminated during harvesting or processing. Gluten free bread can be made from other sources of starch which may include rice flour, potato flour, sorghum flour, corn flour, legumes flour, beans flour, almond flour, etc. These flour do not form elasticity during kneading and therefore guar gum, xantham gum, hydroxypropyle methylcellulose, eggs, corn starch may needed to be added to compensate for gluten protein. These may be helpful in retaining the shape and make bread fluffier.

Gluten is generally regarded as safe and therefore food products containing this may not be notified through systematic labeling procedure. People with gluten sensitivity are unable to metabolize gluten properly and this results in digestive distress. Symptoms of digestive distress may include gas, bloating, diarrhea, constipation or bowel discomfort.

Gluten sensitivity is less severe and digestive symptoms may occur after the intake of gluten and does not appear to have long term effects. A gluten free diet or gluten reduced diet is suggested to prevent the discomfort. There has been misunderstanding among the general public as this diet is being presumed to show a patterns of healthy eating guidelines. It does, but only for the ones who are showing signs and symptoms of gluten sensitivity and not for the general public.

# GLUTEN FREE RECIPES

## 1. Chicken roast

### Ingredients

Chicken quarters 4

Ginger and garlic paste 3 table spoons

Unsweetened yogurt ½ cup

Vinegar ¼ cup

Green chili paste 2 table spoons

Salt and pepper to taste

Sesame seeds oil ¼ cup

### Directions

1. Mix all the ingredients well together and refrigerate for few hours for marinating.
2. Pre-heat oven at medium heat and roast it till it gets tender and attain right color.
3. Serve hot with gluten free sauces and dips of choice.

## 2. Chicken and potato curry

### Ingredients

Chicken with bones small pieces 1 lb.

Potatoes 2 cut in quarters

Onion 3 finely sliced and fried golden brown

Yogurt 1 cup

Red chili powder 1 tea spoon

Ginger and garlic paste 3 table spoons

Coriander seeds powder 1 tea spoon

Cumin seeds powder 1 tea spoon

Five spice powder ½ tea spoon

Green chilies whole 3

Coriander leaves ½ cup chopped

Salt to taste

Oil ½ cup

**Directions**

1. Blend fried onion and yogurt together.
2. Heat oil in a sauce pan and fry chicken with ginger and garlic paste.
3. Add blended ingredients and all the ingredients except coriander leaves.
4. Add four cups of water and bring to boil.
5. Simmer, cover and cook till potatoes and chicken get tender.
6. Remove from stove and add chopped coriander leaves and serve hot with plain rice.

## 3. Baked fish

**Ingredients**

Fish fillet 1 lb.

Coconut cream ½ cup

Lemon juice ¼ cup

Green chili paste 2 table spoons

Salt and pepper to taste

Sesame seed oil ¼ cup

**Directions**

1. Mix together all the ingredients well, cover and keep refrigerated for few hours for marinating.
2. Pre heat oven at medium temperature and bake fish till it gets tender and gain required golden color.
3. Serve hot with salads and plain rice.

## 4. Fried mutton chops

**Ingredients**

Mutton chops 1 lb.

Ginger garlic paste 3 table spoons

Coriander seeds powder 1 tea spoon

Cumin seeds powder 1 tea spoon

Yogurt ¼ cup

Lemon juice 3 table spoon

Raw papaya paste 2 table spoon

Green chili paste 1 table spoon

Garam masala ingredients, cardamom small 4, cloves4, cardamom large 2, cinnamon 1 inch stick 1, mace 1 tea spoon, nutmeg 1/2 tea spoon,  grind all the ingredients in a coffee grinder (use 1 tea spoon of the ground powder for marinating)

Salt and pepper to taste

**Directions**

1.  Mix all the ingredients well together, cover and refrigerate for few hours for marinating.
2.  Deep fry till tender.
3.  Serve hot with salads and plain rice.

## 5. Mutton and spinach curry

**Ingredients**

Mutton leg small pieces 1 lb. wash thoroughly

Spinach 3 cups

Onion 2 sliced

Tomatoes 4 chopped

Ginger and garlic paste 3 table spoons

Cinnamon powder ¼ tea spoon

Mace powder ¼ tea spoon

Nutmeg powder ¼ tea spoon

Salt to taste

Oil ½ cup

**Directions**

1. Fry onion in oil till golden brown.
2. Add chopped tomatoes, ginger and garlic paste and fry.
3. Add mutton and all spices and three cups of water and bring to boil.
4. Simmer, cover and cook on low heat till mutton gets tender.
5. Add spinach and cook uncovered for few minutes.
6. Simmer and cook on low heat for five to ten minutes.
7. Serve hot with rice.

## 6. <u>Coconut fish curry</u>

**Ingredients**

Fish boneless 1 lb. 1 inch cubes

Coconut milk 1 cup

Tomato puree 1 cup

Mustard seeds 1 table spoon

Curry leaves few if available

Fenugreek seed 1 tea spoon

Ginger cloves 6 finely sliced

Salt to taste

Oil ½ cup

**Directions**

1. Fry fish in oil till brown, take it out in a container.
2. In the same oil fry mustard seeds, fenugreek seeds, curry leaves and garlic slice.
3. Add tomato puree, coconut milk, fried fish and salt and simmer, cover and cook for few more minutes.
4. Serve hot with plain rice.

# 7. <u>Chicken kebabs</u>

### <u>Ingredients</u>

Chicken 1 lb. boneless fillet

Onion 2 cut in quarters

Ginger 1 inch piece

Garlic cloves 8

Green chilies 6

Coriander leaves ½ cup

Mint leaves ¼ cup

Lemon juice 2 table spoons

Cumin seeds 1 table spoon

Coriander seeds 1 table spoon

Salt to taste

Oil for shallow frying

### <u>Directions</u>

1. Except oil, chop all the ingredients well in a chopper.
2. Make round disc shaped kebabs between the palms of your hand and shallow fry from both sides till done.
3. Serve hot.

# 8. <u>Beef with okra</u>

### <u>Ingredients</u>

Beef ½ lb. boneless cubes

Onion 2 sliced

Tomatoes 4 chopped

Ginger and garlic paste 2 table spoons

Five spice powder or garam masala powder ½ tea spoon

Red chili powder 1 tea spoon

Okra 2 cups fried

Cumin seeds powder ½ tea spoon

Coriander seeds powder ½ tea spoon

Salt to taste

Oil ½ cup

**Directions**

1. Fry onion slice in oil till golden brown.
2. Add ginger and garlic paste and tomatoes and fry till mushy.
3. Add beef cubes, all spices and enough water needed to make meat tender and for curry.
4. Cover, simmer and cook on low heat till meat gets tender.
5. Add fried okra and cook for few more minutes.
6. Serve hot with rice.

## 9. Chicken fried rice

**Ingredients**

Chicken ½ lb. boneless cubes

Mixed vegetables 3 cups, julienne, carrots, onion, capsicum, spring onion, cabbage

Garlic cloves 8 sliced

Rice 2 cups, long grain basmati, wash and soak for half an hour

Soy sauce ½ cup gluten free

Salt to taste

Oil ½ cup

**Directions**

1. Fry garlic slices in half oil till golden brown.
2. Add chicken cubes and fry till tender.
3. Add vegetable, salt and half soy sauce and fry.
4. Strain out excess water from rice.

5. Add rice and three cups of boiling water, remaining soy sauce, oil and two tea spoons salt and bring to boil.
6. Cover and cook on medium heat till all the water dries.
7. Keep it over pre heated skillet for five to ten more minutes.
8. Uncover rice pan and add fried chicken and vegetables and mix well.
9. Serve hot.

# 10.    Shepherd's pie

## Ingredients

Potatoes 3 boiled and mashed

Beef minced 1 lb.

Onion 2 chopped

Green chilies 3 chopped

Ginger and garlic paste 2 table spoons

Butter 3 table spoon

Milk 1 cup hot

Salt to taste

Black pepper to taste

Oil ¼ cup

## Directions

1. Add butter, salt, pepper and warm milk in mashed potatoes and mix well
2. Fry onion in oil till it softens.
3. Add minced meat, ginger and garlic paste, green chilies, salt and pepper and fry till meat gets tender.
4. In a baking dish evenly spread a layer of mashed potatoes.
5. On top of this layer add minced meat layer.

6. Bake at medium heat in a pre-heated oven for 15-20 minutes or till done.
7. Serve hot.

## 11.    Beef with gram pulse

### Ingredients

Beef 1 lb. boneless cubes

Gram pulses 1 cup wash and soak for one hour

Onion 2 sliced

Garlic and ginger paste 3 table spoons

Tomatoes 4 chopped

Cumin seeds powder 1 tea spoon

Coriander seeds powder 1 tea spoon

Red chili powder 1 tea spoon

Turmeric powder ½ tea spoon

Five spice mix or garam masala powder ½ tea spoon

Coriander leaves ½ cup chopped

Salt to taste

Oil ½ cup

### Directions

1. Fry onion in oil till golden brown.
2. Add tomatoes and ginger and garlic paste and cook till it becomes mushy.
3. Add beef, gram pulse and all the spices and enough water for beef and gram pulse to get tender.
4. Mix well, cover, simmer and cook till meat and gram pulse get tender.
5. Garnish with freshly chopped coriander leaves and enjoy with plain rice.

## 12.    Fried fish

**Ingredients**

Fish fillet 1 lb.

Soy sauce 2 table spoons gluten free

Ginger paste 2 table spoons

Lemon juice 3 table spoons

Coconut cream powder 1 table spoon

3 table spoons

Green chili paste 2 table spoons

Salt to taste

Oil for shallow frying

**Directions**

1. Mix all the ingredients well except oil and marinate fish in the refrigerator for few hours.
2. Shallow fry it from both sides and serve hot with plain rice.

## 13.    Mixed fruit salad

**Ingredients**

Apple 1 diced

Banana1 sliced

Orange 1 sliced

Pear 1 diced

Papaya 1 cup diced

Lemon juice 3 table spoons

Molasses 3 table spoons

Cinnamon powder 1 /4 tea spoon

**Directions**

1. Mix all the ingredients well and serve cold.

## 14.    Chicken with capsicum

**Ingredients**

Chicken 1 lb. small pieces with bones

Capsicum 1 cup diced

Tomatoes 4 chopped

Onion 2 sliced

Ginger and garlic paste 2 table spoons

Five spice mix or garam masala ½ tea spoon

Red chili powder 1 tea spoon

Cumin seeds powder 1 tea spoon

Coriander powder 1 tea spoon

Salt to taste

Oil ½ cup

**Directions**

1. Fry onion till golden brown.
2. Add tomatoes and ginger and garlic paste 3 table spoons and fry till mushy.
3. Add chicken, all the spices and 2 cups of water and mix well. Cover, simmer and cook on low heat till chicken gets tender.
4. Add capsicum and mix well, cover, simmer and cook for five to ten more minutes.
5. Serve hot with rice.

## 15.   Beef and vegetables soup

**Ingredients**

Beef 1cup boneless small cubes

Beef bones 2-3

Garlic 7 cloves whole

Olives 1 cup whole

Mushrooms 1 cup whole

Avocado 1 whole

Onion 1 whole

Tomatoes 4 whole

Coriander leaves 1 cup

Salt and black pepper to taste

Olive oil 3 table spoons

## Directions

1. Boil beef with bones and without bones together in enough water, simmer, cover and cook on low heat till beef gets tender.
2. Mix all the vegetables together and bring to boil, simmer, cover and cook till vegetables get tender.
3. Blend all the vegetables in a blender.
4. Heat oil fry boneless beef pieces till lightly brown.
5. Remove bones and add bone and beef broth to fried beef.
6. Add blended vegetables, mix well and serve hot.

# 16. Sweet and sour chicken

## Ingredients

Chicken 1 cup boneless cubes

Vegetables 1/2 cup slices or cubes each, cabbage, carrots, capsicum, spring onion, onion

Tomato puree 1 cup

Soy sauce ½ cup gluten free

Corn flour ½ cup

Chicken broth 3 cups

Vinegar ¼ cup

Molasses ¼ cup

Green chili chopped 2

Garlic cloves 8 sliced

Salt to taste

Oil ½ cup

### Directions

1.  Fry garlic slice in ¼ cup till golden brown.
2.  Add chicken cubes and fry.
3.  Add vegetables and fry.
4.  In a separate sauce pan fry green chilies and add molasses, vinegar, soy sauce and salt.
5.  Dissolve corn flour in I cup broth and add it to the green chili sauce pan.
6.  Add all the remaining broth and bring it to boil.
7.  Add this sauce to stir fried vegetables and chicken and cook for one more minute on high heat.
8.  Serve hot with rice.

## 17.     Chicken with pineapples

### Ingredients

Chicken 1 cup boneless cubes

Pineapple 1 cup cubes

Onion 1 diced

Capsicum I diced

Garlic 6 cloves sliced

Soy sauce ½ cup gluten free

Vinegar ¼ cup

Chicken broth 1 cup

Corn flour ¼ cup

Salt to taste

Oil ½ cup

### Directions

1.  Fry garlic slice till golden brown.
2.  Add chicken cubes and fry.
3.  Add vegetables and fry.
4.  Add pineapple cubes and remove from heat.

5. Mix together rest of the ingredients and bring it to boil and mix well.
6. Add this sauce to chicken and vegetables stir fry and cook together for one more minute.
7. Serve hot with plain rice.

## 18.    Chicken ginger

### Ingredients

Chicken 1 cup boneless cubes

Tomatoes 3 diced

Onion 1 sliced

Ginger ¼ cup matchsticks

Garlic cloves 6 sliced

Red chili powder ½ tea spoon

All spice powder or garam masala ½ tea spoon

Salt to taste

Oil ½ cup

### Directions

1. Fry garlic slices and onion slices till golden brown.
2. Add chicken cubes and fry.
3. Add tomatoes and spices and fry.
4. Add finely cut ginger over chicken and serve hot.

## 19.    Chicken with almond

### Ingredients

Chicken 1 cup boneless cubes

Almond ½ cup blanched and split into two

Onion 1 diced

Green chilies ½ cup diced, remove seeds

Garlic cloves 10 sliced

Chicken broth 1 cup

Vinegar 2 table spoons

Corn flour ¼ cup

Soy sauce ½ cup gluten free

Salt and pepper to taste

Oil ¼ cup

**Directions**

1. Fry almonds and garlic till golden brown.
2. Add chicken and fry.
3. Add onion and green chilies and fry.
4. In a separate pan prepare sauce by mixing rest of the ingredients.
5. Mix chicken broth with corn flour, vinegar, salt, pepper, soy sauce and bring to boil and mix well.
6. Add it to the chicken and vegetables stir fries.
7. Serve hot with rice.

## 20. Chicken and broccoli with lemon sauce

**Ingredients**

Chicken 1 cup boneless cubes

Broccoli 1 cup cubes

Onion 1 diced

Garlic cloves 8 sliced

Lemon 4 table spoons

Chicken broth 1 cup

Corn flour ¼ cup

Soy sauce ¼ cup gluten free

Salt and pepper to taste

**Directions**

1. Fry garlic slices till golden brown.
2. Add chicken cubes and fry.
3. Add broccoli fry.

4. Add onion and fry.
5. In a separate pan prepare sauce.
6. Mix corn flour with broth, soy sauce, lemon juice, salt and pepper and bring to boil.
7. Add prepared sauce in chicken and vegetables stir fries and cook together for one more minute on high heat.
8. Serve hot with plain rice.

## 21.  Chicken Manchurian

### Ingredients

Chicken 2 cups boneless cubes
Garlic paste 2 table spoons
Green chili paste 1 table spoon
Tomato puree 1 cup
Chicken broth 1-2 cups
Vinegar 1 table spoon
Corn flour ½ cup
Soy sauce ½ cup gluten free
Salt and pepper to taste
Oil ¼ cup

### Directions

1. Mix Chicken cubes with ginger paste, vinegar, green chili paste, soy sauce and corn flour and fry.
2. Add tomato puree, salt, pepper and broth and bring to boil.
3. Cover and simmer for five to ten minutes.
4. Serve hot with rice.

## 22.  Chicken with orange

### Ingredients

Chicken boneless cubes 1 cup

Orange 1 cup cubes

Onion 1 diced

Capsicum 1 diced

Chicken broth 1 cup

Garlic slices 8

Soy sauce ½ cup gluten free

Corn flour ¼ cup

Vinegar 3 table spoons

Salt and pepper to taste

Oil ¼ cup

**Directions**

1. Fry garlic slices till golden brown.
2. Add chicken cubes and fry.
3. Add capsicum and onion and fry.
4. Add orange cubes and move the pan away from stove.
5. Prepare sauce and mix corn flour with broth, vinegar, and soy sauce and bring to boil.
6. Add this prepared sauce to stir fried vegetables and chicken, mix well and cook for one more minute together on high heat.
7. Serve hot with rice.

## 23.     Chicken with spinach

**Ingredients**

Chicken with bones 1 lb.

Spinach 3 cup chopped

Onion 2 sliced

Tomatoes 4 chopped

Ginger and garlic paste 3 table spoons

Red chili powder 1 tea spoon

Coriander seeds powder 1 tea spoon

Cumin seeds powder 1 tea spoon

Turmeric ½ tea spoon

Salt and pepper to taste

Oil ½ cup

### Directions

1. Fry onion till golden brown.
2. Add tomatoes and ginger and garlic paste and fry till it gets mushy.
3. Add chicken and all the spices and fry.
4. Add 2 cups of water and bring to boil.
5. Simmer, cover and cook till chicken gets tender.
6. Add spinach and cook on high heat uncovered for few minutes.
7. Cover, simmer and cook on low heat for five to ten more minutes.
8. Serve hot with rice.

## 24.    Chicken jalfrezy

### Ingredients

Chicken 1 cup boneless cubes

Capsicum 1 cup diced

Cherry tomatoes 1 cup

Onion 1 cup diced

Green chili 1 chopped

Garlic cloves 10

Worcestershire sauce ½ cup

Mustard powder ½ tea spoon

Tomato puree 1 cup

Five spice mix or garam masala powder ½ tea spoon

Black pepper ½ tea spoon

Salt to taste

Oil ½ cup

**Directions**

1. Fry garlic slices till golden brown.
2. Add chicken and fry.
3. Add vegetables and fry.
4. Add rest of the ingredients and mix well.
5. Cook together for few minutes.
6. Serve hot with rice.

## 25. Baked chicken

**Ingredients**

Chicken cut in quarters 4

Yogurt ½ cup

Ginger and garlic paste 3 table spoons

Lemon juice 3 table spoons

Black pepper 1 tea spoon

Salt to taste

Almond powder ½ cup

**Directions**

1. Mix all the ingredients well and keep in the refrigerator for marinating.
2. Pre-heat oven at medium temperature and bake chicken till tender and acquires right color and texture.
3. Serve hot with salads and rice.

## 26. Chicken sash lick

**Ingredients**

Chicken 1 cup boneless cubes

Capsicum 1 cup diced

Tomatoes 1 cup diced

Onion 1 cup diced

Tomato sauce 3 tablespoons

Soy sauce ½ cup gluten free

Garlic paste 1 table spoon

Salt and pepper to taste

Olive oil 1 table spoon

### Directions

1. Mix all the ingredients well and marinade for few hour in the refrigerator.
2. Thread these on skewers alternatingly and grill over charcoal till done.
3. Serve hot with rice.

## 27.  Beef with saffron rice

### Ingredients

Beef 1 lb. boneless cubes

Rice basmati long grains 3 cups wash and soak for half an hour

Onion 2 sliced

Tomatoes 4 chopped

Potatoes 2 cut in quarters and fry

Unsweetened yogurt 1 cup

Ginger and garlic paste 3 table spoons

Garam masala powder or five spice powder 1 tea spoon

Coriander seeds powder 1 tea spoon

Cumin seeds powder 1 tea spoon

Red chili powder 1 tea spoon

Star anise 2

Saffron few strands

Salt to taste

Oil 1 cup

**Directions**

1. Fry onion till golden brown in half of the given oil.
2. Add tomatoes and fry till mushy.
3. Add rest of the ingredients except rice, saffron, potatoes and remaining oil.
4. Add just enough water for the meat to get tender and bring to boil.
5. Cover, simmer and cook till meat gets tender.
6. Dry out any excess water remaining in the beef gravy and make it dry by cooking on high heat and stirring.
7. Drain out excess water from rice and cook it in a wide mouth pan.
8. Add four and a half cups of boiling water, remaining oil, saffron strands and salt to rice and bring it to a boil.
9. Cover and cook rice at medium heat till all the water dries.
10. Keep it over a pre-heated skillet for five to ten more minutes.
11. Take out half of the rice in some container and spread evenly the remaining half in the pan.
12. Pour the gravy layer over the rice layer and the taken out half rice layer over gravy layer. Top it with fried potatoes.
13. Keep over a warm skillet for further ten minutes.
14. Mix well and serve hot.

## 28.    Chicken and chickpea curry

**Ingredients**

Chicken 1 lb. with bones

Chickpeas 1 cup boiled

Onion 1 sliced

Tomatoes 3 chopped

Garlic cloves 8 sliced

Red chili powder 1 tea spoon

Cumin seeds powder 1 tea spoon

Coriander seeds powder 1 tea spoon

Turmeric powder ½ tea spoon

Coriander leaves ½ chopped

Salt to taste

Oil ½ cup

### Directions

1. Fry onion and garlic slices till golden brown.
2. Add tomatoes and fry till mushy.
3. Add chicken and fry.
4. Add chickpeas and spices and fry.
5. Add enough water for chicken to get tender and for required gravy.
6. Cover, simmer and cook till chicken gets tender.
7. Garnish with freshly chopped coriander leaves and serve hot with rice.

## 29.     Chicken saffron rice

### Ingredients

Onion paste ½ cup

Yogurt 1 cup

Chicken 1 cup boneless cubes

Rice 1 cup wash and soak for 30 minutes

Small cardamom 3

Mace powder ¼ tea spoon

Ginger and garlic paste 1 table spoon

Green chili paste 1 table spoon

Saffron few strands

Salt to taste

Oil ½ cup

**Directions**

1. Fry chicken, onion, ginger, garlic, green chili paste for few minutes.
2. Add yogurt, cardamom small, mace powder, saffron strands, rice, salt and two cups of boiling water and bring it to a boil.
3. Cover and cook over medium heat till all the water dries up.
4. Keep the pan over a pre heated skillet for ten more minutes.
5. Mix well and serve hot.

## 30.    Chicken with garlic sauce

**Ingredients**

Chicken 1 cup boneless cubes

Capsicum 1 cup diced

Onion 1 cup diced

Carrots 1 cup diced

Garlic paste 2 table spoon

Vinegar ¼ cup

Chicken broth 2 cups

Corn flour ½ cup

Soy sauce ½ cup gluten free

Salt and pepper to taste

Oil ½ cup

**Directions**

1. Fry chicken in 1 tea spoon garlic paste and ¼ cup of oil.
2. Add onion, capsicum and carrots and fry.

3. Prepare a sauce and in a separate sauce pan fry remaining garlic paste.
4. Dissolve corn flour in chicken broth and add it to the garlic sauce pan.
5. Add vinegar, soy sauce, salt and pepper and bring it to a boil.
6. Add this sauce to chicken and serve hot with plain rice.

# 31. Spicy chicken with mixed vegetables

## Ingredients

Chicken 1 lb. with bones

Onion 2 sliced

Tomatoes 4 chopped

Peas 1 cup

Potatoes 1 cup diced

Carrots 1 cup diced

Garlic 10 cloves sliced

Red chili powder 1 tea spoon

Cardamom small 5 whole Split open

Cinnamon stick 1 inch piece

Cumin seeds powder 1 tea spoon

Salt to taste

Oil ½ cup

## Directions

1. Fry garlic slices and onion in oil till golden brown.
2. Add tomatoes and cook till mushy.
3. Add chicken, spices, salt and two cups water and bring to boil.
4. Mix well, cover, simmer and cook till chicken is half tender.

5. Add vegetables and cook till vegetables and chicken get tender.
6. Serve hot with rice.

## 32.    Egg curry

**Ingredients**

Eggs 6 hard boiled and shelled
Yogurt 1 cup
Onion 2 fried golden brown
Tomatoes 2 chopped
Green chilies 2 chopped
Garlic cloves 8 sliced
Almond powder 2 table spoons
Cumin seeds powder 1 tea spoon
Coriander powder 1 tea spoon
Turmeric powder ½ tea spoon
Cinnamon powder ¼ tea spoon
Fresh coriander leaves ½ cup chopped
Salt to taste
Oil ½ cup

**Directions**

1. In two table spoon of oil fry whole garlic and green chilies.
2. Add chopped tomatoes and fry.
3. In a blender put this fried mixture, fried onion and yogurt and blend well.
4. Now in the same pan pour the remaining oil and fry this blended mixture.
5. Add all the spices and boiled eggs and fry.
6. Add enough water to make gravy of required consistency and bring it to a boil.

7. Mix well, cover, simmer and cook for ten more minutes.
8. Garnish with freshly chopped coriander leaves and serve hot with boiled rice.

# 33.  Eggs and vegetables fried rice

## Ingredients

Eggs 3

Rice 2 cups basmati long grains wash and soak for half an hour

Vegetables ½ cup each diced or julienne, carrots, onion, spring onion, cabbage, capsicum

Soy sauce ½ cup gluten free

Garlic cloves 8 sliced

Salt and pepper to taste

Oil ½ cup

## Directions

1. Drain out excess water from rice.
2. Add three cups of boiling water, two tea spoons salt, ¼ cup soy sauce and ¼ cup oil in rice and cook covered at medium heat till all the water evaporates.
3. Keep rice over pre-heated skillet for five or ten more minutes.
4. Fry garlic slices in little oil till golden brown.
5. Add all the vegetables and remaining soy sauce and fry.
6. Add salt and pepper to taste and mix well and spread these fried vegetables over rice.
7. Fry eggs in little oil and keep mixing so that they are well cooked from all sides.
8. Add little salt and mix now spread cooked eggs over vegetable layer.
9. Mix rice, vegetables and eggs together and serve hot.

## 34.    <u>Scrambled spicy eggs</u>

### <u>Ingredients</u>

Eggs 6

Onion 3 sliced

Tomatoes 4 chopped

Green chilies 3 chopped

Red chili powder 1 tea spoon

Turmeric powder ½ tea spoon

Fresh coriander leaves 1 cup

Salt to taste

Oil ½ cup

### <u>Directions</u>

1.  Fry onion till lightly golden brown.
2.  Add tomatoes and cook till mushy.
3.  Add green chilies, turmeric powder, red chili powder, and salt and mix.
4.  Add eggs and mix well and keep stirring so that eggs are cooked from all sides.
5.  Add chopped coriander leaves and serve hot.

## 35.    <u>Beef with onion</u>

### <u>Ingredients</u>

Beef 1 cup boiled

Onion 1 cup diced

Garlic cloves 6 sliced

Lemon juice 2 table spoons

Oregano 1 table spoon

Salt and black pepper to taste

Oil ½ cup

### <u>Directions</u>

1. Fry garlic slices till golden brown.
2. Add boiled beef and fry.
3. Add onion and fry.
4. Add lemon juice, oregano, salt and pepper and fry.
5. Serve hot with plain rice.

# 36.    Chicken with chilies

## Ingredients

Chicken 1 cup boneless cubes

Onion 1 diced

Garlic cloves 8 sliced

Chicken broth 1 cup

Green chilies ½ cup deseeded cut length wise into two

Soy sauce ¼ cup gluten free

Corn flour ¼ cup

Salt and pepper to taste

## Directions

1. Fry garlic slices in oil till golden brown.
2. Add chicken cubes and fry.
3. Add green chilies and onion and fry.
4. Add soy sauce, salt and pepper.
5. Mix corn flour in chicken broth and add this to chicken and bring it to a boil.
6. Cook for few more minutes and serve hot with plain rice.

# 37.    Beef with chilies

## Ingredients

Beef 1 cup boneless and boiled

Onion 1 cup diced

Green chilies ½ cup deseeded cut length wise into two

Soy sauce ½ cup gluten free

Beef broth 1 cup

Corn flour ¼ cup

Soy sauce ½ cup

Garlic cloves 6 sliced

Salt and pepper to taste

Vinegar 2 table spoons

Oil ½ cup

**Directions**

1. Fry garlic slices till golden brown.
2. Add boiled beef and fry.
3. Add onion and green chilies and fry.
4. Add soy sauce, salt, pepper and vinegar and fry.
5. Mix corn flour in beef broth and add this to the cooking pan and stir well.
6. Bring it to a boil and cook for few more minutes and serve hot.

## 38. Chicken and potato cutlets

**Ingredients**

Chicken 1 cup boiled cubes

Potatoes 3 boiled and mashed

Green chilies 3 chopped

Egg 1 well beaten

Coriander leaves 1 cup chopped

Lemon juice 2 table spoons

Cumin seeds 1 table spoon roasted over a skillet

Salt and pepper to taste

Oil for shallow frying

**Directions**

1. Mix all the ingredients well except oil and egg.

2. Make disc of the mixture with the help of your palms and flatten it to make it half inch thick.
3. Dip in beaten egg and shallow fry from both sides till golden brown.
4. Serve hot.

## 39.    Chicken BBQ

### Ingredients

Chicken 2 lbs. boneless 1 inch cubes
Cream ½ cup
Ginger and garlic paste ¼ cup
Yogurt ½ cup
Green chili paste 2 table spoons
Raw papaya paste 1 table spoon
Red chili powder 1 tea spoon
Cumin seeds powder 1 tea spoon
Coriander seeds powder 1 tea spoon
All spice mix or garam masala powder 1 tea spoon
Salt to taste

### Directions

1. Mix all the ingredients well and marinade for few hour preferably one day in the refrigerator.
2. Thread chicken pieces on skewers and grill over charcoal till done.
3. Serve hot.

## 40.    Beef BBQ

### Ingredients

Beef 2 lb. boneless 1 inch cubes
Yogurt ½ cup
Vinegar ½ cup

Ginger and garlic paste ¼ cup

Meat tenderizer 1 table spoon or raw papaya paste 1 table spoon

Onion paste 1 table spoon

Green chili paste 2 table spoons

Coriander leaves paste 3 table spoons

Cardamom small powder 1 tea spoon

Mace powder ½ tea spoon

Salt to taste

Olive oil 3 table spoons

### Directions

1. Mix all the ingredients well together and keep for marinating in refrigerator for few hours but preferably for one day.
2. Thread beef pieces over skewers and grill over charcoal till done.
3. Serve hot.

## 41.     Chicken BBQ kebabs

### Ingredients

Chicken 2 lb. boneless chunks

Onion 3

Green chilies 5

Ginger 2 inch piece

Garlic cloves 12

Coriander leaves 1 cup

Coriander seeds 1 table spoon roasted over skillet

Cumin seeds 1 table spoon roasted over skillet

Mustard powder 1 tea spoon

Five spice powder or garam masala powder or any spice of choice 1 tea spoon

Yogurt 3 table spoons

Lemon juice 3 table spoons

Salt and pepper to taste

Olive oil 1 table spoon

### Directions

1. Chop all the ingredients well together in a chopper.
2. Spread the chopped mixture with the help of your palms over skewers.
3. Grill over charcoal grill till done.
4. Serve hot.

## 42.     Beef BBQ kebabs

### Ingredients

Beef 2 lb. boneless

Onion 4

Yogurt ¼ cup

Green chilies 5

Coriander leaves 1 cup

Ginger 2 inch piece

Garlic 12 cloves

Coriander seeds 1 table spoon

Cumin seeds 1 table spoon

Five spice mix or garam masala mix or any spice of choice 1 tea spoon

Cream ¼ cup

Corn meal ½ cup

Salt to taste

### Directions

1. Chop all the ingredients well in a chopper.
2. Spread the chopped mixture nicely over skewers with the help of your palm.

3. Grill over charcoal grill till done.
4. Serve hot.

## 43.    Beef steak

### Ingredients

Beef undercut individual pieces 4 pieces

Ginger and garlic paste 1 table spoons

Molasses 1 table spoon

Lemon juice 2 table spoons

Coconut cream powder 1 table spoon

Salt and pepper to taste

Olive oil 3 table spoons

### Directions

1. Marinade beef pieces in all the ingredients listed and keep in the refrigerator for 24 hours.
2. On a grill pan spread out the marinated beef pieces and cover and grill one side till done.
3. Turn it over and cook other half till done.
4. Serve hot with grilled vegetables and mashed potatoes.

## 44.    Chicken steak

### Ingredients

Chicken 4 steak pieces

Ginger paste 1 table spoon

Green chili paste 1 table spoon

Lemon juice 2 table spoon

Red chili powder 1 tea spoon

Cumin seeds powder 1 tea spoon

Honey 1 table spoon

Yogurt 4 table spoons

Tomato sauce 1 table spoon

Salt and pepper to taste

Butter melted 3 table spoons

**Directions**

1. Marinade chicken pieces for at least 24 hour in all the listed ingredients and keep it cold in the refrigerator.
2. Spread chicken pieces over grill pan evenly and grill on both sides evenly and keep covered while cooking to reduce moisture loss during cooking.
3. Serve hot with grilled vegetables and mashed potatoes.

## 45.    Beef and gram pulses curry

**Ingredients**

Beef 1 lb. boneless pieces

Gram pulses 1 cup wash and soak for one hour

Onion 2 sliced

Tomatoes 4 chopped

Ginger and garlic paste 2 table spoons

Cinnamon stick 1 inch piece

Cloves 4

Cardamom small 4

Cumin seeds powder 1 table spoon

Red chili powder 1 tea spoon

Salt and pepper to taste

Coriander leaves ½ cup chopped

Oil ½ cup

**Directions**

1. Fry onion slices and whole spices in oil till golden brown.
2. Add ginger and garlic paste and tomatoes and fry till mushy.
3. Add all the remaining ingredients and fry.

4. Add enough water for meat and gram pulses to get tender.
5. Mix well, cover, simmer and cook till meat and gram pulses get tender.
6. Garnish with freshly chopped coriander leaves and serve hot with rice or corn bread.

## 46. Chicken with tomatoes

### Ingredients

Chicken 1 lb. boneless pieces
Tomatoes 6 chopped
Green chilies 8 chopped deseed if you want less hot
Ginger and garlic paste 2 table spoons
Coriander leaves 1 cup chopped
Turmeric powder ½ tea spoon
Salt to taste
Five spice powder or garam masala powder 1 tea spoon
Oil ½ cup

### Directions

1. Fry chicken with ginger and garlic paste.
2. Add tomatoes and fry till tomatoes are mushy.
3. Add 1 cup water bring to boil, cover and simmer.
4. When half tender, add green chilies, cover and cook till tender.
5. Add chopped coriander leaves and fry for few minutes.
6. Serve hot with rice.

## 47. Minced beef with capsicum

### Ingredients

Beef minced 1 lb.
Capsicum 2 diced

Onion 2 sliced

Tomatoes 4 chopped

Ginger and garlic paste 3 table spoons

Cumin seeds powder 1 table spoon

Turmeric powder ½ tea spoon

Coriander powder 1 tea spoon

Red chili powder 1 tea spoon

Cardamom small 6

Salt to taste

Oil ½ cup

**Directions**

1. Fry onion and cardamom small till golden brown.
2. Add tomatoes and ginger and garlic paste and cook till mushy.
3. Add minced meat and all the spices and fry.
4. Add capsicum and fry.
5. Serve hot.

## 48. <u>Chicken with capsicum</u>

**Ingredients**

Chicken 1 lb. boneless pieces

Tomatoes 4 chopped

Onion 2 sliced

Ginger and garlic paste 2 table spoons

Cumin seeds powder 1 table spoon

Capsicum 2 diced

Red chili powder 1 tea spoon

Salt to taste

Oil ½ cup

**Directions**

1. Fry onion slices till golden brown.

2. Add tomatoes, ginger and garlic paste, chicken, cumin seeds powder, red chili powder and salt and fry.
3. Add one cup of water and bring to boil.
4. Mix well, cover, simmer and cook till tender.
5. Add diced capsicum and fry, simmer and let it cook for few more minutes.
6. Serve hot.

## 49.   Mined beef with potatoes

### Ingredients

Beef minced 1 lb.

Potatoes 3 diced

Onion 2 sliced

Tomatoes 4 chopped

Cardamom small 5

Ginger and garlic paste 3 table spoons

Green chili paste 2 table spoons

Cloves 4

Cinnamon stick 1 inch piece

Cumin seeds powder 1 table spoon

Turmeric powder ½ tea spoon

Yogurt ½ cup

Coriander leaves ½ cup chopped

Salt to taste

Oil ½ cup

### Directions

1. Fry onion and cardamom till onion turns golden brown.
2. Add tomatoes, green chili paste, ginger and garlic paste, salt and fry till tomatoes are mushy.
3. Add minced meat, yogurt, salt and all the spices and fry.
4. Add potatoes and one cup of water and bring to boil.

5. Mix well, cover, simmer and cook till potatoes get tender.
6. Garnish coriander leaves and serve hot.

# 50.     <u>Mutton and potato curry</u>

## Ingredients

Mutton 1 lb. leg pieces

Potatoes 3 cut in quarters

Onion 2 sliced and fried till golden brown

Tomatoes 2 chopped

Yogurt 1 cup

Small cardamoms 6 split them open

Cloves 5

Cinnamon stick 1 inch piece

Ginger and garlic paste 3 table spoons

Red chili powder 1 tea spoon

Cumin seed powder 1 table spoon

Turmeric powder ½ tea spoon

Salt to taste

Fresh coriander leaves ½ cup chopped

Oil ½ cup

## Directions

1. Fry mutton with ginger and garlic paste and whole spices.
2. Add tomatoes and fry till tomatoes get mushy.
3. Add rest of the spices and enough water for meat to get tender.
4. Mix well, cover, simmer, and cook till meat is almost done.
5. Blend yogurt with fried onions and 1 cup water.

6. Add blended mixture and potatoes and salt to the mutton pan and cook till potatoes get tender.
7. Garnish with freshly chopped coriander leaves and serve hot with rice.

## 51.    Minced beef and spinach

### Ingredients

Beef minced 1 lb.

Spinach 3 cups

Onion 2 sliced

Tomatoes 4 chopped

Ginger and garlic paste 3 table spoons

Yogurt ½ cup

Whole spices of choice, cardamom small, cloves, cinnamon stick, 1 table spoon

Red chili powder 1 tea spoon

Cumin seeds powder 1 table spoon

Salt to taste

Oil ½ cup

### Directions

1. Fry onion slices with whole spices till onion turns golden brown.
2. Add tomatoes, ginger and garlic paste and fry till mushy.
3. Add minced beef, yogurt and rest of the ingredients and keep frying for few more minutes.
4. Add 1 cup water and bring to boil.
5. Mix well, cover, simmer and cook for ten to fifteen more minutes.
6. Serve hot with rice.

## 52.    Minced beef with peas

### Ingredients

Beef minced 1 lb.

Peas 1 cups

Onion 2 sliced

Tomatoes 4 chopped

Ginger and garlic paste 2 table spoons

Yogurt ½ cup

Whole spices of choice 1 table spoon

Cumin seeds powder 1 table spoon

Red chili powder 1 tea spoon

Salt to taste

Oil ½ cup

### Directions

1. Fry onion and whole spices till onion turns golden brown.
2. Add tomatoes and ginger and garlic paste till tomatoes get mushy.
3. Add yogurt, minced meat, peas and rest of the ingredients and 1 cup water and mix well and bring to boil.
4. Cover, simmer and cook for fifteen minutes.
5. Uncover and fry for few more minutes.
6. Serve hot.

## 53.     Chicken, peas and potato rice

### Ingredients

Chicken 1 cup boneless cubes

Peas 1 cup

Potatoes 1 cup diced

Onion 1 sliced

Tomatoes 3 chopped

Red chili powder 1 tea spoon

Cumin seeds powder 1 tea spoon

Garlic clove 6 sliced

Salt to taste

Oil ½ cup

**Directions**

1. Fry onion and garlic in oil till they become golden brown.
2. Add tomatoes and fry till mushy.
3. Add chicken and fry.
4. Add peas, potatoes, spices and 1 cup water and bring to boil.
5. Mix well, cover, simmer and cook on low heat till potatoes get tender.
6. Serve hot with rice.

## 54.    Chicken salad

**Ingredients**

Chicken boneless cubes 1 cup

Carrots 1 cup boiled

Potatoes 1 cup boiled

Peas 1 cup boiled

Cream cheese ½ cup

Coconut cream ½ cup

Honey 2 table spoon

Salt and pepper to taste

Sesame seeds oil 3 table spoons

**Directions**

1. Fry chicken in little oil till golden brown.
2. Mix all the ingredients well in a mixing bowl and serve cold.

## 55.     Beef salad

### Ingredients

Beef 1 cup boneless small cubes boiled and fried

Corn 1 cup

Potatoes 1 cup boiled

Chickpeas 1 cup boiled

Red beans 1 cup boiled

Mustard sauce 1 table spoon roasted over skillet

Olive oil 3 table spoons

Lemon juice 2 table spoons

Salt and pepper to taste

### Directions

1.   Mix all the ingredients well and serve cold.

## 56.     Chicken and vegetables soup

### Ingredients

Chicken 1 cup boneless cubes

Quinoa 1 cup boiled

Mixed vegetables 1 cup

Garlic 6 cloves

Tomatoes 3

Onion 1

Salt and pepper to taste

Olive oil 3 table spoon

### Directions

1.   Mix all the ingredients and cook in enough water to make soup.
2.   Blend all the ingredients well in a blender.
3.   Bring it to a boil and add more water if needed.
4.   Cook for ten more minutes and serve hot with gluten free croutons.

## 57.    Beef with mixed vegetables soup

**Ingredients**

Beef 1 cup cubes

Mixed lentils ½ cup

Tomatoes 4

Potato 1

Onion 1

Coriander leaves 1 cup

Olives ½ cup

Salt and pepper to taste

**Directions**

1. Mix all the ingredients and cook in enough water till tender.
2. Blend all the ingredients well in a blender.
3. Bring it to a boil and add more water if needed.
4. Cook for ten more minutes and serve hot.

## 58.    Chicken with baby corns

**Ingredients**

Chicken 1 cup boneless cubes

Baby corn 1 cup

Cherry tomatoes 1 cup

Baby onion 1 cup

Lemon juice 2 table spoons

Mustard powder ½ tea spoon

Garlic 6 cloves sliced

Worcestershire sauce ½ cup

Salt and pepper to taste

Oil ½ cup

**Directions**

1. Fry garlic slices till golden brown.
2. Add chicken cubes and fry.
3. Add onion and baby corn and fry.
4. Add cherry tomatoes and fry.
5. Add rest of the ingredients, cover and fry for five more minutes.
6. Serve hot.

## 59.      Chicken with mushrooms

### Ingredients

Chicken 1 cup boneless cubes

Mushrooms 1 cup sliced

Almond milk 1 cup

Garlic cloves 6 sliced

Lemon juice 2 table spoons

Salt and pepper to taste

### Directions

1. Fry garlic slices till golden brown.
2. Add chicken and fry.
3. Add mushrooms and fry.
4. Add rest of the ingredients and cook covered for five more minutes.
5. Serve hot.

## 60.      Beef with lentils

### Ingredients

Beef 1 cup boneless cubes

Mixed lentils 1 cup

Onion 1 sliced

Tomatoes 3 chopped

Ginger and garlic paste 2 table spoons

Herbs and spices of choice 1 table spoon

Salt and pepper to taste

Oil ½ cup

**Directions**

1. Fry garlic and onion till golden brown.
2. Add tomatoes and ginger and garlic paste and fry till mushy.
3. Add rest of the ingredients and 3 cups of water and cook till tender.
4. Serve hot with rice.

# 61.    Creamy chicken pasta

**Ingredients**

Chicken 1 cup boneless cubes

Gluten free pasta 3 cups boiled and strained

Avocado 1 peeled and sliced

Onion 1 diced

Garlic cloves 8 sliced

Cream cheese 1 cup

Tomato puree 1 cup

Basil 1 table spoon

Worcestershire sauce 3 table spoons

Salt and pepper to taste

Oil ½ cup

**Directions**

1. Fry garlic in oil till golden brown.
2. Add chicken cubes and fry.
3. Add Worcestershire sauce and fry.
4. Add diced onion and fry.
5. Add avocado slices and fry.
6. Add rest of the ingredients.

7. Mix well, cover, simmer and cook for five more minutes.
8. Serve hot.

## 62.    Baked beef pasta

### Ingredients

Beef 1 cup boneless cubes boiled
Onion 1 cup diced
Mushrooms 1 cup sliced
Parsley 1 table spoon
Garlic cloves 6 sliced
Corn meal ½ cup
Gluten free pasta of choice 3 cups boiled and strained
Milk 1-2 cups
Lemon juice 3 table spoons
Salt and pepper to taste
Olive oil ½ cup

### Directions

1. Fry garlic in half oil till golden brown
2. Add boiled beef and fry.
3. Add onions and mushrooms and fry.
4. In a separate sauce pan fry corn meal in remaining oil for few minutes.
5. Add milk slowly stirring continuously so that lumps are not formed.
6. Add salt, pepper and parsley and mix well.
7. Add this sauce to beef stir fry and add all the remaining ingredients.
8. Mix well, cover, simmer and cook together for five more minutes.
9. Serve hot.

# 63.    Sweet and sour spaghetti

### Ingredients

Beef minced 1 cup

Capsicum 1 cup chopped

Garlic cloves 8 sliced

Onion 1 cup chopped

Tomatoes 1 cup chopped

Lemon juice 4 table spoons

Honey 4 table spoons

Cilantro 1 table spoon

Gluten free spaghetti 3 cups boiled and strained

Beef broth 1 cup

Salt and pepper to taste

Olive oil ½ cup

### Directions

1. Fry garlic slices in oil till golden brown.
2. Add onion and fry.
3. Add tomatoes and fry till mushy.
4. Add minced meat and fry.
5. Add rest of the ingredients.
6. Mix well, cover, simmer and cook together for five more minutes.
7. Serve hot.

# 64.    Gluten-free tortillas

### Ingredients

Rice powder 2 cups

Corn meal 2 cups

Corn flour 1 cup

Egg 2

Cumin seeds powder 1 table spoon

Cilantro 1 table spoon

Salt and pepper to taste

Oil ½ cup

### Directions

1. Except oil mix all the ingredients well together and knead (use milk if needed).
2. Using rolling pin and board roll it using little dry corn meal for easy rolling.
3. Cook it over pre-heated skillet and spread oil on each side with the help of a spoon.
4. Serve hot.

## 65.　　Potato tortillas

### Ingredients

Potatoes 5 boiled and mashed

Corn flour 2 cups

Coriander leaves fresh 1 cup chopped

Red chili powder 1 tea spoon

Mustard seeds 1 table spoon

Salt and pepper to taste

Oil ½ cup

### Directions

1. Mix all the ingredients well and knead (if required add some milk).
2. Using rolling pin and board roll it to make a tortilla using little extra corn flour if needed.
3. Cook it over a pre heated skillet and turn over to make sure it is cooked from all sides.
4. Spread oil on both sides while cooking.
5. Serve hot.

## 66.     Corn and egg tortillas

### Ingredients

Corn meal 4 cups

Eggs 2

Green chilies 2 chopped

Garlic paste 1 table spoon

Salt and pepper to taste

Oil ½ cup

### Directions

1. Mix all the ingredients together and knead (use milk or extra corn meal if needed).
2. Roll it using a rolling pin and board.
3. Cook it over a pre-heated skillet turning over and cooking from all sides.
4. Spread oil on both sides.
5. Serve hot.

## 67.     Creamy tomato and egg soup

### Ingredients

Tomatoes 8 chopped

Onion 2 chopped

Coriander leaves 1 cup chopped

Egg 1 well beaten

Garlic 5 cloves

Vinegar 2 table spoons

Molasses 2 table spoons

Fresh cream ½ cup

Salt and pepper to taste

Olive oil ½ cup

### Directions

1. In oil fry all the vegetables.

2. Add enough water and all the ingredients except egg and cream and cook till tender.
3. Blend all together.
4. Bring to boil and add more water if needed.
5. Add well beaten and stir quickly.
6. Add cream and mix.
7. Serve hot.

# 68. Chicken and mushroom soup

### Ingredients

Chicken 1cup boneless chopped

Mushrooms 2 cups sliced

Onion 1 chopped

Garlic cloves 6 chopped

Corn flour 1 cup

Chicken broth 4-6 cups

Soy sauce ½ cup gluten free

Vinegar 3 table spoons

Salt and pepper to taste

Sesame seeds oil 4 table spoons

### Directions

1. Fry garlic in oil and add chopped chicken and fry.
2. Add mushrooms and onion and fry.
3. Dissolve corn flour in broth and add rest of the ingredients and bring to boil and cook together for few minutes.
4. Serve hot.

# 69. Corn and chicken rice

### Ingredients

Chicken 1 cup boneless cubes

Corn 1 cup

Rice 2 cups basmati long grain, wash and soak in water

Garlic cloves 7 sliced

Onion 1 chopped

Tomatoes 3 chopped

Green chili paste 1 table spoon

Salt and pepper to taste

Oil ½ cup

**Directions**

1. Fry garlic in oil till golden brown.
2. Add onion and fry.
3. Add chicken and fry.
4. Add corn and fry.
5. Add rest of the ingredients and 3 cups of boiling water.
6. Mix well, cover, simmer and cook till rice get dry.
7. Keep the pan over pre-heated skillet for five to ten more minutes.
8. Serve hot.

## 70.    Fried chicken

**Ingredients**

Chicken 1lb. with bones and skin

Rice flour ½ cup

Corn flour ½ cup

Gram flour ½ cup

Ginger and garlic paste 2 table spoons

Vinegar 3 table spoons

Cumin seeds powder 1 table spoon

Green chili paste 1 table spoon

Salt and pepper to taste

Oil for deep frying

### Directions

1. Mix salt, pepper, rice flour, corn flour and gram flour and keep aside for chicken coating.
2. Marinade chicken in rest of the ingredients except oil for few hours.
3. Press each chicken piece on dry coating and coat it properly from all sides.
4. Fry each piece till golden brown.
5. Serve hot.

## 71.    Chicken and tomato curry

### Ingredients

Chicken 1 lb. small pieces with bones

Tomatoes 6 grill over grill pan

Green chilies 4 grill over grill pan

Curry leaves few if available

Garlic 8 cloves grill over grill pan

Onion 1 grill over grill pan

Sesame seeds 3 table spoons roasted over skillet

Yogurt ½ cup

Red chili powder 1 tea spoon

Coriander seeds powder 1 tea spoon

Cumin seeds powder 1 tea spoon

Coriander leaves ½ cup chopped

Salt to taste

Oil ½ cup

### Directions

1. Blend all the grilled and roasted ingredients well in a blender.
2. Marinade chicken in yogurt, red chili powder, cumin seeds powder, coriander seeds powder for some time.

3. Fry chicken and add blended mixture.
4. Mix well, cover, simmer and add enough water to make gravy.
5. Cook till chicken gets tender.
6. Garnish with freshly chopped coriander leaves and serve hot with rice.

## 72.    Chicken green curry

### Ingredients

Chicken 1 lb. small pieces with bones

Coconut powder 3 table spoons

Garlic cloves 8

Green chilies 6

Coriander leaves 1 cup

Cumin seeds powder 1 table spoon

Salt and pepper to taste

Pea nuts ¼ cup roasted peanut powder

Oil ½ cup

### Directions

1. Blend together green chilies, coriander leaves, garlic, cumin seeds, coconut powder in little water.
2. Fry this blended mixture with chicken.
3. Add rest of the ingredients and fry.
4. Add enough water to make gravy.
5. Mix well, cover, simmer and cook till chicken gets tender.
6. Serve hot with rice.

## 73.    Chicken coconut curry

### Ingredients

Chicken boneless cubes 1 cup

Coconut milk 1 cup

Tomato puree 1 cup

Ginger and garlic paste 1 table spoon

Green chili paste 1 table spoon

Cumin seeds powder 1 table spoon

Coriander leaves ½ cup chopped

Salt to taste

Oil ½ cup

**Direction**

1. Fry chicken with ginger and garlic paste and green chili paste
2. Add rest of the ingredients and fry.
3. Add enough water to make gravy.
4. Mix well, cover, simmer and cook till tender.
5. Garnish with freshly chopped coriander leaves and serve hot with rice.

## 74. Grilled chicken with vegetables

**Ingredients**

Chicken 4 boneless large chunks

Vegetables mixed 1 cup of choice, add 1 table spoon vinegar and little salt and pepper

Honey 2 table spoons

Ginger paste 2 table spoons

Yogurt ¼ cup

Lemon juice 2 table spoon

Almond powder 2 table spoon

Salt and pepper to taste

Oil 4 table spoon

**Directions**

1. Except vegetables mix all the ingredients well and keep in the refrigerator for marinating for some time.
2. Grill these chicken pieces over a grill pan on both sides.
3. Grill the vegetables and serve hot together.

## 75. Roast chicken with stir fried vegetables

### Ingredients

Chicken quarters 4

Mixed vegetables of choice 2-4 cups

Yogurt ½ cup

Lemon juice 4 table spoons

Green chili paste 2 table spoons

Molasses 1 table spoon

Ginger and garlic paste 2 table spoons

Mustard powder 1 tea spoon

White pepper 1 tea spoon

Salt to taste

Oil 3 table spoons

### Directions

1. Mix all the ingredients together except vegetables and oil.
2. Keep chicken in the refrigerator for marinating.
3. Roast chicken in the pre-heated oven till done.
4. Stir fry vegetables in oil and little salt and pepper.
5. Serve hot.

## 76. Minced meat and potato cutlet

### Ingredients

Minced meat 1 cup

Potatoes 4 boiled and mashed

Onion 1 chopped

Green chilies 3 chopped

Coriander leaves 1 cup chopped

Egg 1 well beaten

Salt and pepper to taste

Oil for shallow frying

**Directions**

1. Fry onion in little oil till soft.
2. Add minced meat and fry.
3. Add green chilies and fry
4. Add this fried minced meat to mashed potatoes and mix.
5. Add coriander leaves, salt and pepper and mix well.
6. Take a handful and make a round cutlet of the mixture.
7. Dip it in well beaten egg and shallow fry from both sides till golden brown in a pre-heated fry pan of oil.
8. Serve hot.

## 77.    Spicy prawn rice

**Ingredients**

Prawn 1 cup de veined

Rice 2 cups, wash and soak for 30 minutes

Green chili paste 1 table spoon

Tomato puree ½ cup

Coconut milk ½ cup

Ginger and garlic paste 1 table spoon

Red chili powder 1 tea spoon

Coriander leaves ½ cup chopped

Cumin seeds powder 1 tea spoon

Salt to taste

Oil ½ cup

**Directions**

1. Fry prawns in ginger and garlic paste and green chili paste till done.
2. Add rest of the ingredients and three cups of boiling water.
3. Mix well, cover, simmer and cook till done.
4. Keep the pan over pre heated skillet for five to ten minutes.
5. Serve hot.

## 78.     Sweet and sour prawns

### Ingredients

Prawns 1 cup
Egg 1 well beaten
Corn flour ¾ cup
Soy sauce ½ cup gluten free
Tomato sauce ½ cup
Honey 4 table spoon
Vinegar 3 table spoon
Mixed vegetables 1 cup diced, onion, carrots, capsicum
Garlic paste 1 table spoon
Salt and pepper to taste
Oil ½ cup

### Directions

1. Add ½ cup corn flour, garlic paste, little salt, little pepper, 2 table spoons soy sauce in well beaten egg and mix well.
2. Marinade prawns in egg mixture for some time.
3. Deep fry prawns till done.
4. Fry vegetables in oil and add fried prawns.
5. Make a sauce by mixing rest of the ingredients and little water and bring it to a boil.

6. Add this prepared sauce to vegetables and prawns and mix well and serve hot with rice.

# 79. Chicken spicy BBQ

### Ingredients

Chicken quarters 4

Yogurt ¼ cup

Lemon juice 4 table spoons

Green chili paste 2 table spoons

Ginger and garlic paste 2 table spoons

Cumin seeds powder 1 table spoon

Coriander seeds powder 1 tea spoon

Mace powder ¼ tea spoon

Salt and pepper to taste

Sesame seeds oil 2 table spoons

### Directions

1. Mix all the ingredients well and marinade chicken in the mix for few hours.
2. Use skewers to fasten chicken pieces and grill over charcoal from all sides till done.
3. Serve hot.

# 80. Mutton BBQ chops

### Ingredients

Mutton chops 1 lb.

Five spice mix 1 tea spoon

Vinegar ¼ cup

Ginger and garlic paste 3 table spoons

Yogurt ¼ cup

Raw papaya paste or meat tenderizer 1 table spoon

Salt to taste

**Directions**

1. Marinade mutton in the listed ingredients for some time.
2. Thread mutton chops over skewers and grill over charcoal till done.
3. Serve hot.

# 81.    <u>Chicken gluten-free pizza</u>

**Ingredients**

Corn meal ½ cup

Rice flour ½ cup

Potato flour ½ cup

Yeast 1 table spoon

Egg 1

Milk ¼ cup warm

Butter 1 table spoon

Sugar 1 tea spoon

Salt to taste

Fried chicken chunks 1 cup

Mixed vegetables 1 cup

Cheese shredded 1 cup

Pizza sauce ½ cup

**Directions**

1. Except last four listed ingredients knead all the ingredients together well and keep it covered at a warm place for some time to rise.
2. Pre heat oven at medium heat.
3. Spread the kneaded mixture with the help of your hands over a pizza baking tray.
4. Spread pizza sauce over it.
5. Spread selected diced vegetables over it.
6. Spread chicken chunks over it.

7. Spread shredded cheese over it.
8. Bake it for 10-15 minutes or till done.
9. Serve hot.

# 82. Mutton grilled chops

## Ingredients

Mutton chops 1 lb.

Onion paste 1 table spoon

Green chili paste 1 table spoon

Ginger and garlic paste 2 table spoons

Yogurt ¼ cup

Lemon juice 2 table spoons

Raw papaya paste 1 table spoon

Red chili powder 1 tea spoon

Cumin seeds powder 1 table spoon

Salt and pepper to taste

Oil 2 table spoons

## Directions

1. Marinade mutton in the listed ingredients for few hours.
2. Grill these over grill pan on both sides till done.
3. Serve hot.

# 83. Mutton roast

## Ingredients

Mutton leg small 1

Ginger and garlic paste 3 table spoons

Yogurt ½ cup

Vinegar ½ cup

Five spice powder or garam masala powder 1 tea spoon

Raw papaya paste 2 table spoons

Green chili paste 2 table spoons

Salt to taste

Oil 2 table spoons

**Directions**

1. Marinade mutton leg in all the listed ingredients for 24 hours.
2. Roast it in a pre-heated oven till done.
3. Serve hot.

## 84. Mutton and potato curry

**Ingredients**

Mutton 1 lb. leg pieces small

Onion 2 sliced

Tomatoes 4 chopped

Ginger and garlic paste 3 table spoons

Potatoes 2 cut in quarters

Red chili powder 1 tea spoon

Coriander seeds powder 1 tea spoon

Five spice powder or garam masala powder 1 tea spoon

Salt to taste

Oil ½ cup

**Directions**

1. Fry onion in oil till golden brown.
2. Add tomatoes and ginger and garlic paste and fry till mushy.
3. Add rest of the ingredients except potatoes and fry for five minutes.
4. Add enough water for mutton to get tender, cover, simmer and cook till half tender.
5. When half cooked, add potatoes, cover, simmer and cook till tender.
6. Add extra water to make gravy and bring it to a boil.

7. Simmer and cook for ten more minutes.
8. Serve hot with rice.

# 85.   **Mutton and okra curry**

### Ingredients

Mutton leg 1 lb. small pieces

Okra ½ lb. fried in little oil

Onion 2 sliced

Tomatoes 4 chopped

Ginger and garlic paste 2 table spoons

Red chili powder 1 tea spoon

Cumin seeds powder 1 tea spoon

Coriander powder 1 tea spoon

Five spice powder or garam masala powder ½ tea spoon

Coriander leaves ½ cup chopped

Salt to taste

Oil ½ cup

### Directions

1. Fry onion till golden brown.
2. Add chopped tomatoes and ginger and garlic paste and fry till mushy.
3. Add mutton and rest of the ingredients except okra and fry.
4. Add enough water for meat to get tender, mix well, cover, simmer and cook till tender.
5. Add fried okra and mix.
6. Add chopped coriander and serve hot with rice.

# 86.   **Mutton with mixed vegetables**

### Ingredients

Mutton leg 1 lb. small pieces

Onion 1 sliced

Ginger and garlic paste 2 table spoons

Yogurt ½ cup

Tomatoes 2 chopped

Salt to taste

Herbs and spices according to choice

Vegetables mixed 2 cups of choice

Oil ½ cup

### Directions

1. Fry onion till golden brown.
2. Add mutton and yogurt and fry.
3. Add rest of the ingredients except vegetables and fry.
4. Add enough water for meat to get tender and cook on low heat till meat gets tender.
5. Add vegetables and cook for ten more minutes.
6. Serve hot.

## 87.    Mutton spicy rice

### Ingredients

Mutton leg 1 lb. small pieces

Yogurt 1 cup

Onion 1 sliced

Green chili paste 2 table spoons

Tomatoes 3 chopped

Ginger and garlic paste 2 table spoons

Whole spices 1 table spoon, small cardamom, large cardamom, cloves, cinnamon, bay leaf, star anise

Rice 3 cups long grains basmati wash and soak for 30 minutes

Salt to taste

Oil ½ cup

### Directions
1. Fry onion and whole spices in oil till onion turns golden brown in color.
2. Add tomatoes, ginger and garlic paste and green chili paste and fry.
3. Add mutton and yogurt and fry.
4. Add enough water for meat to get tender and cook on low heat.
5. Add rest of the ingredients, four and a half cups of boiling water and mix well, cover and cook on medium heat till dry.
6. Keep it over a pre heated skillet for five to ten more minutes.
7. Serve hot.

## 88.    Minced meat Pizza

### Ingredients
Beef minced 1 cup

Onion 1 chopped

Garlic paste 1 table spoon

Mixed vegetables of choice 1 cup

Pizza sauce ½ cup

Cheese 1 cup shredded

Salt and pepper to taste

Corn flour ½ cup

Rice flour ½ cup

Tapioca flour ½ cup

Yeast 1 table spoon

Sugar 1 tea spoon

Egg 1 well beaten

Butter 1 table spoon

Milk 1/4 cup warm

**Directions**

1. Mix eight last listed ingredients together and keep in a warm place to rise.
2. Fry onion in oil till tender.
3. Add Minced beef, garlic paste, salt and pepper and mix well and fry.
4. Spread pizza dough over a pizza tray evenly.
5. Spread pizza sauce over it.
6. Add minced meat and cheese.
7. Add mixed vegetables and bake in a pre-heated oven for 10-15 minutes or till done.
8. Serve hot.

## 89.  Mutton BBQ

**Ingredients**

Mutton 1 lb. leg pieces small

Ginger and garlic paste 2 table spoons

Onion paste 2 table spoons

Green chili paste 2 table spoons

Cumin seeds powder 1 table spoon

Yogurt ¼ cup

Raw papaya paste or meat tenderizer 1 table spoon

Vinegar 3 table spoons

Salt and pepper to taste

**Directions**

1. Thread mutton pieces over skewers and grill over charcoal till done.
2. Serve hot.

## 90.  Mutton green coconut curry

**Ingredients**

Mutton leg 1 lb. small pieces

Coconut milk 1 cup

Green chilies 5

Coriander leaves 1 cup

Cumin seeds 1 table spoon

Onion 1

Garlic cloves 12

Salt and pepper to taste

Yogurt 1 cup

Oil ½ cup

**Directions**

1. Blend green chilies, onion, coriander leaves, garlic, and cumin seeds in a little water.
2. Fry mutton in oil and blended mixture for few minutes.
3. Add rest of the ingredients and mix well.
4. Add enough water to make gravy and to make meat tender.
5. Cover, simmer and cook till tender.
6. Serve hot with rice.

# 91.  **Mutton jalfrezy**

**Ingredients**

Mutton leg 1 lb. small pieces

Tomato puree 1 cup

Capsicum 1 cup diced

Cherry tomatoes 1 cup whole

Onion 1 cup diced

Worcestershire sauce ½ cup

Mustard powder ½ tea spoon

Five spice powder or garam masala powder ½ tea spoon

Cumin seeds powder ½ tea spoon

Coriander seeds powder ½ tea spoon

Garlic cloves 12 sliced

Salt and black pepper to taste

Oil ½ cup

**Directions**

1. Fry garlic slices till golden brown in half oil.
2. Add mutton and fry.
3. Add rest of the ingredients except vegetables.
4. Add enough water for meat to get tender.
5. Mix well, cover, simmer and cook on low heat till meat gets tender.
6. Fry vegetables in a separate fryer in remaining oil.
7. Add these to mutton, mix well and cook together for few more minutes.
8. Serve hot.

# 92.  Mutton ginger

**Ingredients**

Mutton leg 1 lb. small pieces

Onion2 sliced

Ginger ½ cup finely chopped

Tomatoes 4 chopped

Green chili paste 1 table spoon

Coriander seeds powder ½ tea spoon

Cumin seeds powder ½ tea spoon

Turmeric powder ½ tea spoon

Five spice powder or garam masala powder ½ tea spoon

Salt to taste

Oil ½ cup

**Directions**

1. Fry onion in oil till golden brown.
2. Add tomatoes and green chili paste and fry.
3. Add mutton and fry.
4. Add rest of the ingredients except ginger and fry.
5. Add enough water for meat to get tender, mix well, simmer, cover and cook on low heat till meat gets tender.
6. Add finely chopped ginger and serve hot with rice.

## 93.   Mutton BBQ kebab

### Ingredients

Mutton leg 1 lb. small pieces

Yogurt ¼ cup

Lemon juice 3 table spoons

Paprika 1 table spoon

Cilantro 1 table spoon

Meat tenderizer 1 tea spoon

Ginger powder 1 table spoon

White pepper 1 tea spoon

Salt to taste

### Directions

1. Marinade mutton in all the listed ingredients for 24 hours.
2. Thread mutton pieces over skewers and grill over charcoal till done.
3. Serve hot.

## 94.   Mutton with peas

### Ingredients

Mutton leg 1 lb. small pieces

Onion 1 sliced

Peas 1 cup

Tomatoes 4 chopped

Ginger and garlic paste 2 table spoons

Five spice powder or garam masala powder½ tea spoon

Red chili powder 1 tea spoon

Cumin seeds powder 1 tea spoon

Coriander seeds powder 1 tea spoon

Turmeric powder ½ tea spoon

Salt to taste

Oil ½ cup

### Directions

1. Fry onion in oil till golden brown.
2. Add tomatoes and cook till mushy.
3. Add rest of the ingredients except peas and fry.
4. Add enough water for meat to get tender and to have enough gravy.
5. Add peas and cook for five to ten more minutes.
6. Serve hot with rice.

## 95. Mutton with capsicum

### Ingredients

Mutton leg 1 lb. small pieces

Capsicum 1 cup diced

Onion 1 sliced

Tomatoes 3 chopped

Ginger and garlic paste 2 table spoons

Herbs and spices of choice

Salt to taste

Oil ½ cup

### Directions

1. Fry onion in oil till golden brown.
2. Add tomatoes and fry till mushy.

3. Add rest of the ingredients except capsicum and fry.
4. Add enough water needed to get mutton tender.
5. Add capsicum and cook for few more minutes.
6. Serve hot with rice.

## 96. Mutton and almond curry

### Ingredients

Mutton leg 1 lb. small pieces

Onion 2 fried golden brown

Yogurt 1 cup

Almonds ½ cup blanched and roasted

Cilantro 1 table spoon

Green chili 1

Ginger I inch piece

Garlic Cloves 8

Salt and pepper to taste

Herbs and spices of choice 1 table spoon

Oil ½ cup

### Directions

1. Blend fried onion with yogurt, ginger, garlic, cilantro and almonds.
2. Add these to a pan and fry.
3. Add mutton and fry.
4. Add rest of the ingredients and enough water for meat to get tender.
5. Mix well, cover, simmer and cook on low heat till mutton gets tender.
6. Serve hot with rice.

## 97. Mutton fried rice

### Ingredients

Mutton leg 1 lb. small pieces

Rice 3 cups long grain basmati wash and soak for 30 minutes

Onion 3

Green chili 3

Ginger 1 inch piece

Garlic 12 cloves

Cardamom small 12

Cloves 12

Black pepper whole 15

Yogurt 1 cup

Mace powder ¼ tea spoon

Nutmeg powder ¼ tea spoon

Black pepper powder ½ tea spoon

Oil ½ cup

**Directions**

1. Blend onion, ginger, garlic, green chilies and yogurt with little water.
2. Fry mutton in oil with whole spices for few minutes.
3. Add blended mixture and fry.
4. Add enough water for meat to get tender.
5. Mix well, simmer, cover and cook on low heat till mutton gets tender.
6. Add rice and four cups of boiling water and cover and cook on medium heat till dry.
7. Keep it over and pre-heated skillet for five to ten more minutes
8. Sprinkle top with black pepper powder, nutmeg powder, mace powder and mix well.
9. Serve hot.

## 98.    Baked mutton

### Ingredients

Mutton leg 1 lb. small pieces boiled

Onion 2 diced

Tomatoes 4 diced

Coconut milk 1 cup

Capsicum 1 diced

Herbs and spices of choice mix 1 table spoon

Salt to taste

Oil ½ cup

### Directions

1. Mix all the ingredients and bake in a pre-heated oven for 30 minutes or till done.
2. Serve hot with rice.

## 99.    Mutton fry

### Ingredients

Mutton leg 1 lb. small pieces

Onion 3 slices

Red chilies pepper whole 4

Vinegar ¼ cup

Black cumin seeds 1 table spoon

Ginger and garlic paste 2 table spoons

Salt to taste

Oil ½ cup

### Directions

1. Fry onion till golden brown.
2. Add rest of the ingredients and mix well.
3. Add enough water and cook till tender.
4. Fry for few more minutes and serve hot with rice.

## 100.    Mutton with mushrooms

## Ingredients

Mutton leg 1 lb. small pieces

Tomatoes 4 chopped

Onion 2 sliced

Mushrooms 1 cup diced and fried

Soy sauce ½ cup gluten free

Salt and pepper to taste

Oil ½ cup

Directions

1. Fry onion in oil till golden brown.
2. Add tomatoes and fry.
3. Add mutton and fry.
4. Add rest of the ingredients except mushrooms and fry.
5. Add enough water to make the meat tender.
6. Add fried mushrooms, mix well and serve hot with rice.

www.ingramcontent.com/pod-product-compliance
Lightning Source LLC
Chambersburg PA
CBHW070123290526
45789CB00005B/2121